Table of Contents

OVERVIEW

Leukemia is a cancer of the blood cells. There are several broad categories of blood cells, including red blood cells (RBCs), white blood cells (WBCs), and platelets. Generally, leukemia refers to cancers of the WBCs.

WBCs are a vital part of your immune system. They protect your body from invasion by bacteria, viruses, and fungi, as well as from abnormal cells and other foreign substances. In leukemia, the WBCs don't function like normal WBCs. They can also divide too quickly and eventually crowd out normal cells.

WBCs are mostly produced in the bone marrow, but certain types of WBCs are also made in the lymph nodes, spleen, and thymus gland. Once formed, WBCs circulate throughout your body in your blood and lymph (fluid that circulates through the lymphatic system), concentrating in the lymph nodes and spleen.

LUEKEMIA DIET RECIPES

BREAKFAST

1. Persimmon and Date Cobbler

Prep Time: 35 minutes

Cook Time: 40 minutes

Total Time: 1 hour 15 minutes

Makes: about 9 servings

Ingredients

- 1 cup peeled and chopped fuyu persimmons (typically 1-2 pieces of fruit)
- 1/3 cup chopped Medjool dates
- 1/2 cup orange juice (Water is fine, too, but orange juice adds a delightful 'je nais se quoi!')
- 2 cups granulated sugar (separated in to 1 cup portions)
- 1 teaspoon vanilla
- 1 cup all-purpose flour
- 1/2 teaspoon salt
- 2 teaspoons baking powder

- 1/2 cup buttermilk (Kefir or whole milk can be substituted)
- 1/4 cup salted butter, melted
- Optional: Salted caramel ice cream

Directions:

1. Preheat oven to 375 degrees F.
2. Add the first three ingredients in to a bowl and mix with 1 cup sugar and vanilla
3. In another bowl, combine the remaining cup of sugar, flour, salt, and baking powder. Add the buttermilk to the batter and stir to blend.
4. Put the melted butter in the bottom of the baking pan.
5. Pour batter in to the pan.
6. Stir the fruit/sugar mixture and pour atop the batter.
7. Bake on the middle oven rack for 50 minutes - 1 hour, or until the crust resembles a golden brown hue, similar in color to honey.
8. Serve warm with an optional scoop of salted caramel ice cream.

2. Mexican Green Chile + Potato Pancakes

Prep Time: 15 miuntes

Cook Time: 25 miuntes

Total Time: 40 miuntes

Makes about 12 Servings

Ingredients:

- 1 tablespoon butter
- 1/4 cup green onions, chopped (from about 2 green onions)
- 1/2 cup sweet white onion (Maui or Vidalia), chopped
- 1/4 cup Hatch green chiles, chopped (such as these)
- 1 large russet potato, skinned and cut in half (try to find a potato that is 3/4-1 lb.)
- 1/4 teaspoon garlic powder
- 1/4 teaspoon freshly-ground black pepper
- 1/2 teaspoon salt
- 1 1/4 teaspoon baking powder
- 1/4 cup flour
- 1 egg, beaten
- (Optional) Sour cream and jalapeno pepper jelly (such as this)

Directions:

1. In a small sauté pan, melt butter over medium-high heat.

2. Add green and white onions and season with salt and freshly-ground black pepper, to taste.

3. Sauté for 3 minutes.

4. Add green chiles and continue to sauté for about 5 more minutes.

5. Remove from heat and set aside.

6. Add water about 1/3-1/2 way up a large mixing bowl.

7. Using the box grater, grate the potatoes and put the flesh into the large mixing bowl filled with water. Set aside.

8. In a small bowl, combine the dry ingredients (garlic powder, pepper, salt, baking powder, flour) and set aside.

9. In another small bowl, add the egg and beat until combined. Set aside.

10. Cover a cookie sheet with paper towels and set near the stove.

11. Fill a large sauté pan about 1/4-1/3 of the way high with vegetable oil. Turn heat to medium (it will take a few minutes for the oil to warm).

12. Place the colander in the sink and drain the potatoes.

13. Using a light tea towel or cheesecloth, add the potatoes like a bundle and squeeze out as much excess water as you can.

14. Put potatoes back into the large mixing bowl. Add the onion/green chile mixture - dry ingredients - and beaten egg. Stir to combine.

15. Bring mixture over to the stove. Turn heat to medium-high.

16. Using a tablespoon (or a larger slotted spoon, depending on your desired size), add pancake mix one

by one to the hot oil. Note that cooking time for each side of the pancake could take up to 3-minutes!

17. Place finished pancakes on a paper towel-lined cookie sheet to cool.

18. Repeat until all pancakes have been made.

19. Serve warm with optional sour cream and jalapeno jelly.

3. Summer Cherry Cobbler

Prep Time: 10 minutes

Cook Time: 35 minutes

Total Time: 45 minutes

Makes about 9 servings

Ingredients:

- *1 14.5-ounce can red tart cherries in water (I use this brand)
- 2 cups granulated sugar (separated in to 1 cup portions)
- 1 teaspoon vanilla
- 1 cup all-purpose flour
- 1/2 teaspoon salt
- 2 teaspoons baking powder
- 1/2 cup whole milk
- 1/4 cup salted butter, melted
- Optional: Salted caramel ice cream

Directions:

1. Preheat oven to 375 degrees F.

2. Pour entire can of cherries (juice included) in to a
   bowl and mix with 1 cup sugar and vanilla

3. In another bowl, combine the remaining cup of sugar,
   flour, salt, and baking powder. Add the whole milk to
   the batter and stir to blend.

4. Put the melted butter in the bottom of the baking pan.

5. Pour batter in to the pan.

6. Stir the cherry/sugar mixture and pour atop the
   batter.

7. Bake on the middle oven rack for 50 minutes - 1 hour,
   or until the crust resembles a golden brown hue,
   similar in color to honey.

8. Serve warm with an optional scoop of salted caramel
   ice cream.

4. Homemade Pizza Sauce

Prep Time: 10 minutes

Cook Time: 25 minutes

Total Time: 35 minutes

Make about: 8 to 12 servings

Ingredients:

- 1/2 T EVOO (extra virgin olive oil)
- 1 clove garlic, minced
- 1 14.5-ounce can crushed tomatoes (I prefer the Italian San Marzano variety)
- 1/3 c broth (chicken or vegetable)
- 1/2 t dried oregano
- 1/2 t dried basil
- 1 t salt
- Freshly ground black pepper, to taste
- Optional: 3 T fresh basil chiffonade

Directions

1. In a saucepan, add oil and allow to get warm over medium-high heat

2. Add garlic and saute for 30 seconds (you don't want the garlic to get brown and toasty)

3. Add remainder of ingredients up to the optional basil chiffonade and bring to a boil

4. Cover and simmer on low for 30 minutes

5. Remove from heat and season to taste

6. Optional: When room temperature, add basil chiffonade

5. Crisp & Buttery Pan Pizza

Prep Time: 15 minutes

Cook Time: 35 mintes

Total Time: 50 minutes

Makes about: 9 servings

Ingredients:

- 2 cups all-purpose flour
- 1 teaspoons fine salt (table salt or fine sea salt)
- 1/2 teaspoon instant yeast or active dry yeast
- 3/4 cups lukewarm water
- 1 tablespoon olive oil plus 1 1/2 tablespoons olive oil for the pan
- 6 ounces low-moisture mozzarella, grated (about 1 1/4 cups, loosely packed)
- 1/2 cup pizza sauce, homemade or store-bought

Directions:

1. Weigh your flour, or measure it by gently spooning it into the cup, then sweeping off any excess.

2. Place the flour, salt, yeast, water, and 1 tablespoon of the olive oil in the bowl medium-large mixing bowl.

3. Stir everything together to make a shaggy, sticky mass of dough with no dry patches of flour. This should take about 1 minute by hand, using a spoon or spatula. Scrape down the sides of the bowl to gather the dough into a rough ball, then cover the bowl.

4. After 5 minutes, uncover the bowl and reach a bowl scraper or your wet hand down between the side of the bowl and the dough, as though you were going to lift the dough out. Instead of lifting, stretch the bottom of the dough up and over its top. Repeat three more times, turning the bowl 90 degrees each time. This process of four stretches, which takes the place of kneading, is called a fold.

5. Re-cover the bowl, and after 5 minutes do another fold. Wait 5 minutes and repeat, then another 5 minutes and do a fourth and final fold. Cover the bowl and let the dough rest, undisturbed, for 40 minutes. Then refrigerate it for a minimum of 12 hours, or up to 72 hours. It'll rise slowly as it chills, developing

flavor; this long rise will also add flexibility to your schedule.

6. At least 3 hours before you want to serve your pizza, prepare your pan. Pour 1 1/2 tablespoons olive oil into your 9-10 inch oven-safe heavy-bottomed skillet of similar size, or a 10-inch round cake pan or 9-inch square pan. Tilt the pan to spread the oil across the bottom, and use your fingers or a paper towel to spread some oil up the edges, as well.

7. Transfer the dough to the pan and turn it once to coat both sides with the oil. After coating the dough in oil, press the dough to the edges of the pan, dimpling it using the tips of your fingers in the process. The dough may start to resist and shrink back—that's okay, just cover it and let it rest for about 15 minutes, then repeat the dimpling and pressing. At this point the dough should reach the edges of the pan—if it doesn't, give it one more 15-minute rest before dimpling and pressing a third and final time.

8. Cover the crust and let it rise for 2 hours at room temperature. The fully risen dough will look soft and pillowy (your dough will resemble the photo, below).

9. About 30 minutes before baking, place one rack at the bottom of the oven and one toward the top (about 4 to 5 inches from the top heating element). Heat the oven to 450°F.

10. When you're ready to bake the pizza, sprinkle about three-quarters of the mozzarella (a scant 1 cup) evenly over the crust. Cover the entire crust, no bare dough showing—this will yield caramelized edges. Dollop small spoonfuls of the sauce over the cheese (don't spread it!)—laying the cheese down first like this will prevent the sauce from seeping into the crust and making it soggy. Sprinkle on the remaining mozzarella and optional toppings.

11. Bake the pizza on the bottom rack of the oven for 18 to 20 minutes, until the cheese is bubbling and the bottom and edges of the crust are a rich golden brown (use a spatula to check the bottom). If the bottom is brown but the top still seems pale, transfer the pizza to the top rack and bake for 2 to 4 minutes longer. On the other hand, if the top seems fine but the bottom's not browned to your liking, leave the pizza on the

bottom rack for another 2 to 4 minutes. Home ovens can vary a lot, so use the visual cues and your own preferences to gauge when you've achieved the perfect bake.

12. Remove the pizza from the oven. Sprinkle with the optional Parmesan cheese and garlic powder, dried oregano, and hot pepper flakes.

13. Place the pan on a heatproof surface. Carefully run a table knife or spatula between the edge of the pizza and side of the pan to prevent the cheese from sticking as it cools. Let the pizza cool very briefly, then as soon as you feel comfortable doing so, carefully transfer it from the pan to a cooling rack or cutting surface. This will prevent the crust from becoming soggy.

6. Braised Beef with Dried Cherries

Prep Time:10 minutes

Cook Time: 45 minutes

Total Time: 55 minutes

Make about: 4 servings

Ingredients:

- 2 T all-purpose flour
- 1 t ground black pepper
- 2 t kosher salt
- 1 lb beef stew meat, cut in to 3-in cubes
- 1/4 c EVOO (extra virgin olive oil)
- 1 large sweet white onion, peeled and chopped
- 4 cloves garlic, peeled and chopped
- 1 c red wine
- 1 c dried cherries
- 3 c beef stock
- 2 bay leaves
- Pinch of dry thyme or 2 sprigs of fresh thyme
- Optional: 2 T corn starch

Directions:

1. Place pot over medium-high heat and add oil. Allow to get hot!

2. Pat off any excess flour on beef and, working in batches, brown beef on all sides, apprx. 30 seconds/side. Set beef aside.

3. Add onions to the pot and season with a generous pinch each of salt and pepper. Saute for 3 minutes.

4. Add garlic (to the onions) and continue to saute for another minute.

5. Add red wine and stir to combine (onions and garlic). Allow the wine to reduce by half (this took apprx. 4 minutes).

6. Add beef stock, beef, cherries, bay leaves and thyme. Bring to a boil, then reduce to a low simmer and cover.

7. Set timer for 3 hours, checking back a few times to stir.

8. Remove bay leaves (and thyme sprigs if you used fresh).

9. Season with salt and pepper, to taste.

Optional step: If you feel like the broth is too runny, follow the below steps to thicken:

1. Remove the beef from the liquid and set aside momentarily.

2. In a small dish or mug, combine 1 T of corn starch with 1 T of water and stir vigorously to combine.

3. While stirring the hot liquid in the pot, slowly pour the corn starch/water mixture in to the liquid and keep stirring for a few moments to ensure that it has been evenly distributed.

4. Should you feel that the broth still isn't thick enough, repeat above steps 2 and 3 again.

5. Add the beef back to the liquid.

7. Savory Heirloom Tomato Pie

Prep Time: 10 minutes

Coook Time: 25 minutes

Total Time: 35 minutes

Makes about: 8 servings

Ingredients:

- 3/4 cup grated Parmigiano-Reggiano cheese, broken out by 1/4 cup and 1/2 cup
- 2 1/4 pounds (36 ounces) assorted heirloom tomatoes, thinly sliced (if you can't find heirloom tomatoes, any large red tomatoes will do)
- 1 tbsp. olive oil
- 1 cup sweet white onion, chopped
- 1/2 cup freshly grated Gruyere cheese
- 1/4 cup mayonnaise
- 1/4 cup Ranch dressing
- 1/8 teaspoon freshly-ground black pepper (if you don't have 1/8 teaspoon, use a heavy pinch)
- 1/3 cup chopped fresh chives

- 1/3 cup chopped fresh arugula (you can also combine this with fresh basil or even cilantro - whatever herbs you have on-hand!)
- Salt and pepper, to taste

Directions:

1. Bake the pre-made pie dough/your homemade dough according to the directions. Remove from oven and sprinkle 1/4 cup of grated Parmigiano-Reggiano cheese on the bottom of the crust.

2. Set aside to cool.

3. Pre-heat oven to 350 F.

4. Cover the surface of a large cookie sheet with paper towels and top with a layer of sliced tomatoes. Sprinkle with salt. Place single layer of paper towels atop the tomatoes and repeat the previous step until all sliced tomatoes have been placed atop paper towels and salted. (This will literally resemble a "paper towel and tomato" lasagna.) Let stand for at least 30

minutes (up to 1 hour) while you prep the rest of your ingredients.

5. Over medium heat, heat oil and add the chopped onion, plus a liberal sprinkle of salt and freshly-ground black pepper. Saute until tender, approximately 5-7 minutes. Remove from heat and set aside.

6. Combine the remainder of the cheeses (1/2 cup each Parmigiano-Reggiano and Gruyere), plus mayonnaise, Ranch dressing, and 1/8 teaspoon freshly-ground black pepper in a small bowl and set aside.

7. Combine the herbs (chopped chives and arugula/mix) in a bowl. *Reserve one teaspoon of this herb blend for later and set aside.

8. Add sauteed onions to the bowl of herbs and stir to combine.

9. Assemble your work-space: Pie crust, tomatoes, herb/onion mix.

10. Layer tomatoes and the herbs/onion mix in the prepared crust, repeating until you have relinquished your ingredients. You will likely have 3-5 layers.

11. Pour the cheese/mayo/Ranch mixture atop the pie and, with a gentle hand, evenly-spread across the perimeter.

12. If your pie crust has edges, shield them with foil to prevent further browning/cooking. Bake at 350 F for 45 minutes (on the middle rack, or one approx. 5" from oven ceiling) or until topping is lightly browned.

13. Remove the pie from the oven and discard the foil surrounding the edges.

14. Optional: To further brown the top, set oven to broil and return the pie to the same rack. Broil for 1-2

minutes or until the topping becomes golden brown and bubbly.

15. Remove from the oven and sprinkle the pie with the reserved teaspoon of herbs. Serve hot, warm, room-temp, or cold! You simply cannot go wrong here, folks!

8. Maple-Roasted Whole Carrots

Prep Time: 15 minutes

Cook Time: 40 minutes

Total Time: 55 minutes

Make about: 6 servings

Ingredients:

- 1 bunch organic carrots (if you can, choose rainbow over orange - they're so pretty!)
- 1 tbsp. coconut oil
- 1 tbsp. Dijon or whole-grain mustard
- 1 tbsp. maple syrup
- Salt and pepper, to taste

Directions:

1. Preheat oven to 400 degrees F

2. Scrub carrots thoroughly to remove dirt - pat dry. Remove the top stem and the bottom nib (do not worry about peeling).

3. In a small cup, mix coconut oil, mustard, and maple syrup together. Pour in to a pan that's large enough to fit the carrots, length-wise.

4. Add carrots to the pan and toss to evenly distribute mixture.

5. On a baking sheet lined with foil or parchment paper (I prefer the latter), lay carrots and season with salt and pepper, to taste. Set pan with remaining mixture aside.

6. Roast for 20 minutes. Remove from the oven and flip the carrots over. Re-season with salt and pepper, to taste.

7. Roast for 25 more minutes or until tender with the pierce of a fork or sharp knife.

8. Remove from oven. Add carrots back to the pan with the remaining coconut oil/mustard/syrup mixture and gently toss to evenly distribute.

9. Serve immediately, or allow to cool and enjoy later as
    a side dish or chopped for a great salad topper!

9. The Best Banana Bread You've Never Had

Prep Time: 15 minutes

Cook Time: 30 minutes

Total Time: 45 minutes

Make about: 8 servings

Ingredients:

- stick salted butter, melted and cooled
- 1 1/4 cups all-purpose flour
- 3/4 cup granulated sugar
- 1 teaspoon baking powder
- 1 teaspoon salt
- 1/2 teaspoon baking soda
- 1/2 teaspoon ground cinnamon
- 2/3 cup dark chocolate chips
- 2/3 cup butterscotch chips
- 2 large eggs
- 1/2 cup full fat sour cream OR yogurt
- 1 teaspoon vanilla extract
- 1 cup mashed ripe banana (approximately two bananas)

Directions

1. Preheat oven to 350 degrees F

2. Using a pastry brush, lightly butter one 9-by-5-inch loaf pan

3. Whisk the flour, granulated sugar, baking powder, salt, baking soda, and cinnamon in a large bowl. Add both the chocolate and butterscotch chips.

4. Whisk the eggs, 1/2 cup cooled melted butter, sour cream or yogurt, and vanilla in a medium bowl. Stir in the mashed banana. Fold the banana mixture into the flour mixture until just combined.

5. Spread the batter in to the prepared pan. Bake until a toothpick inserted into the center comes out clean, about 60-65 minutes.

6. Using a toothpick/cake tester, gently prick holes in to the cake with about 1/2-3/4 insertion.

7. Reheat the remaining cooled melted butter, approximately 10 seconds. Evenly pour the remaining melted butter atop the cake, allowing for it to penetrate in the pricked holes.

8. Enjoy warm or seal tightly and nosh later!

10. Dump Cake

Prep Time: 20 minutes

Cook Time: 25 minutes

Total Time: 45 minutes

Make about: 12 servings

Ingredients:

- 1 can (21 oz.) cherry pie filling
- 1 can (15 oz.) crushed pineapple, liquid drained
- 1 box (18 oz.) yellow cake mix
- 1/3 cup oats
- 2 sticks (8 oz.) butter, sliced
- Note: I use salted butter.
- *Optional: Vanilla bean ice cream

Directions:

1. In a 13x9" baking dish, dump cherry pie filling and liquid-drained crushed pineapple. Stir together.

2. Dump the cake mix and oats on top of fruit filling, and spread evenly. Top with sliced butter, distributed evenly

3. Bake at 400-degrees for 45-50 minutes; until topping is a rich, golden brown.

4. Serve warm with a scoop of vanilla-bean ice cream!

11. Andrew & Bronson's Cheese Bread

Prep Time: 15 minutes

Cook Time: 25 minutes

Total Time: 40 minutes

Make about: 8 servings

Ingredients:

- 1 ¾ cups all-purpose flour
- 1 tablespoon baking powder
- 1 teaspoon salt
- ¼ teaspoon white pepper
- pinch of cayenne pepper
- 3 large eggs, at room temperature
- 1/3 cup whole milk, at room temperature
- 1/3 cup extra virgin olive oil
- 1 generous cup of grated gruyere
- 2.5 ounces white cheddar, cut into very small cubes
- ¾ cup thinly sliced scallions

Directions:

1. Preheat oven to 350 degrees F. Butter loaf pan.

2. Whisk flour, baking powder, salt and white pepper together in a large bowl.

3. In a separate bowl add eggs and whisk for one minute. Whisk in milk and olive oil.

4. Combine wet ingredients to the dry ingredients using a sturdy wooden spoon or rubber spatula. Do not overwork the dough – beating the dough too much will toughen the consistency of the bread.

5. Stir in cheeses and scallions. Turn the dough into the buttered loaf pan. Pat the top of the dough with the back of the spatula or spoon in the pan to even it out.

6. Bake for 35 – 45 minutes, or until the bread has become golden.

7. Once baked, transfer the pan to a cooling rack, and let cool for five minutes or so. Run a knife along the edges to loosen the bread from the pan.

8. Turn the loaf over to release it on to the rack. Invert and cool right side up.

12. Southern-style green bean casserole

Prep Time: 5 minutes

Cook Time: 15 minutes

Total Time: 20 minutes

Make about: 10 servings

Ingredients:

- 2-16 oz. bags of French-cut string beans

Chef's note: Cook the green beans on the stove according to the package directions but, instead of water, use chicken broth to enhance the flavor. Drain the beans after cooking.

- 1 10.5 oz. can Cream of Mushroom soup
- 8 oz. sour cream
- 6 slices of Kraft Deli Deluxe American Cheese Singles
- 1/2 cup crushed Ritz Crackers
- 3 tablespoons salted butter, cut in to dice-sized cubes

Directions:

1. Spray non-stick cooking spray in an 11x7 glass baking pan.

2. In a separate bowl, combine the first three ingredients and stir to blend. Season, to taste, with salt and freshly-ground black pepper.

3. Pour in to glass pan.

4. Cover evenly with cheese slices, so mixture underneath is not visible.

5. Evenly top with Ritz Cracker crumbs.

6. To finish, dot the top of the casserole with cubed butter.

7. Bake, uncovered, at 325 degrees for 30-minutes.

13. Los Cabos-inspired chilaquiles

Prep Time: 5 minutes

Cook Time: 15 minutes

Total Time: 20 minutes

Make about: 1 servings

Ingredients:

- 3 corn tortillas
- 1/4 cup vegetable oil
- 1/4 cup chopped sweet white-onion, such as Maui or Vidalia
- 1/2 cup shredded mild-cheddar or Monterrey Jack cheese
- 1/2 cup of red or green enchilada sauce - or your favorite salsa
- 2 tablespoons of chicken or vegetable broth
- 3/4 or 1 cup of cooked and shredded chicken, preferably white breast meat
- 1 egg

Directions:

1. In a small saucepan, add oil and warm over medium heat, approximately 2-minutes.

2. One at a time, add corn tortillas to oil, allowing a 30-second simmer on each side, using tongs to flip.

3. Remove tortilla from oil, and place on paper-towel-topped plate.

4. Repeat until all tortillas have been cooked in oil. Set aside.

5. In a small bowl, combine enchilada sauce or salsa and chicken/vegetable broth and stir. Pour sauce on to a clean dinner plate.

6. One at a time, dip each side of the tortilla in to the sauce, remove, then set aside. Each tortilla should be moist, but not dredged.

7. Using your hands, or a knife, rip each tortilla in to ample bite-sized pieces, keeping each pile separated (thus 3 piles). Set aside.

8. Evenly disperse approximately one-teaspoon of the sauce in to the bottom of the oven-proof French onion

soup bowl.   This will prevent the tortillas from sticking to the bottom of the bowl, thus making clean-up a bit easier!

9. Next, evenly disperse the torn shreds from one tortilla atop the teaspoon of sauce.

10. Top the tortilla shreds with the following ingredients, packing with light force: 1 tablespoon chopped onion (optional), 1/4 cup shredded chicken (optional), 2-tablespoons shredded cheese, and 2-tablespoons of sauce. This process is similar to making lasagna.

11. Repeat until all tortillas, cheese, onions and chicken have been used. Pour remaining sauce on top of the casserole.

12. Line a cookie sheet with foil then place constructed bowl atop. There should be approximately 1/4' of room left in the bowl, from the top of the ingredients to the rim of the bowl. If not, pack with gentle force.

13. *Optional step: As if you were making a sunny-side-up egg, crack egg on top of casserole; do not attempt to scramble.

14. Bake in a 425-degree oven for 13-14 minutes. Enjoy!

15. "Cool Ranch" Saltine Crackers

Prep Time: 5 minutes

Cook Time: 15 minutes

Total Time: 20 minutes

Make about: 4 serving

- 1 1/2 boxes of Multigrain Saltine Crackers (6 sleeves, total)
- 2 cups canola oil
- 2 1-ounce packages of Ranch dressing mix
- 1/4 cup crushed red pepper

Directions:

1. In a small bowl, combine canola oil, Ranch dressing mix, and crushed red pepper. Whisk until blended and set aside.

2. Gently empty cracker sleeves in to a 1-gallon plastic bag, such as Ziploc.

3. Pour wet mixture over the crackers - seal bag - then gently shake to distribute ingredients.

4. For even distribution, lightly toss cracker bag (no need to open the bag) every 15-minutes, for approximately 1 hour.

5. Set bag aside, and allow to sit overnight.

16. Chile-con-Queso

Prep Time: 20 minutes

Cook Time: 35 minutes

Total Time: 55 minutes

Make about: 6 servings

Ingredients:

- 3/4 cup chopped white onion
- 2 tablespoons vegetable oil or butter
- 4 4-ounce cans chopped green chile
- 1/4 cup finely chopped cilantro
- Pinch of garlic powder
- 1/2 cup chicken (or vegetable) broth
- 3/4 cup crushed tomatoes (or Rotel)
- 4-ounces medium sharp cheddar cheese, cubed
- 16-ounces Monterrey Jack cheese, cubed
- 4-ounces cream cheese
- 16 oz. Velveeta cheese, cubed
- 1/2 cup canned evaporated milk or sour cream
- Large cooking pot

Directions:

1. In a large cooking pot, add 2 tablespoons of corn oil and allow to warm for 2 minutes over medium heat.

2. Drop 3/4 cup of chopped white onion in to pot and stir frequently until they become almost translucent. Season lightly with salt and pepper.

3. Next, add green chile, cilantro, pinch of garlic powder, chicken/vegetable broth and crushed tomatoes/Rotel.

4. Stir ingredients together then place lid 3/4 way shut over the pot.

5. Simmer on low heat for 30 minutes, stirring occasionally.

6. Next, remove lid and add all cheeses and canned milk/or sour cream.

7. Turn heat back up to medium and stir frequently until all cheese is melted. Season to taste.

8. Serve with tortilla chips, Fritos, or fresh tortillas and enjoys

17. "White trash" Ambrosia

Prep Time: 2 hours

Cook Time: 0

Total Time: 2 hours

Make about: 15 servings

Ingredients:

- 1 20oz. can crushed pineapple, with juice
- 1/3 cup chopped pistachios
- 1 box (3.4oz) JELL-O Pistachio Flavor Instant Pudding
- 12 oz. whipped cream
- 1 bag (10.5 oz) miniature marshmallows
- 12 oz. cottage cheese
- 2 drops of green food coloring

Directions:

1. In a large mixing bowl, combine all ingredients.

2. Stir until everything is evenly blended/distributed.
3. Refrigerate for 24-hours prior to serving.

18. Turkish Red Lentil Soup

Prep Time: 30 minutes

Cook Time: 7 minutes

Total Time: 37 minutes

Make about: 5 servings

Ingredients:

- 1 tablespoon olive oil
- 1 large sweet white onion (Vidalia and Maui are my favorite sweet varieties), chopped
- 2 garlic cloves, minced
- 1 tablespoon tomato paste
- 1 teaspoon cumin
- 1/2 teaspoon kosher salt
- 1/2 teaspoon black pepper
- Pinch of ground chili powder
- 1 quart plus 2 cups chicken broth (Want to make it vegetarian? Sub the chicken broth for vegetable broth!)
- 1 cup red lentils
- 1 large carrot, peeled and diced
- Juice of 1/2 lemon

- 3 tablespoons chopped fresh mint (cilantro or arugula will also do!)

Directions:

1. In a large pot, heat oil over high heat until hot and shimmering. Add onion and garlic, and sauté until golden, about 7 minutes.

2. Stir in tomato paste, cumin, salt, black pepper and chili powder; sauté for 2 minutes longer.

3. Add broth, lentils and carrot. Bring to a simmer, then partially cover pot and turn heat to medium-low. Simmer until lentils are soft, about 30 minutes. Taste and add salt if necessary.

4. Using an immersion or regular blender or a food processor, puree half the soup then add it back to the pot. Soup should be somewhat chunky.

5. Stir in lemon juice and chopped greens.

19. Coca-Cola Brownie Cake

Prep Time: 15 minutes

Cook Time: 30 minutes

Total Time: 45 minutes

Make about: 10 to 15 servings

Ingredient:

Cake

- 2 cups sugar
- 2 cups all purpose flour
- 1 1/2 cups small marshmallows
- 1/2 cup salted butter
- 1/2 cup vegetable oil
- 3 tablespoons cocoa (I swear by Hershey's)
- 1 cup Coca-Cola
- 1 teaspoon baking soda
- 1/2 cup buttermilk
- 2 eggs
- 1 teaspoon vanilla extract

Icing

- 3/4 cup salted butter

- 4 1/2 tablespoons cocoa

- 9 tablespoons Coca-Cola

- 24 ounces (3 cups) confectioner's sugar (a.k.a. powdered sugar)

- 1 1/2 teaspoons vanilla extrac

Directions:

Cake

1. Preheat oven to 350 degrees.

2. In a bowl, combine: sugar, flour and marshmallows.

3. In a saucepan, add: butter, oil, cocoa and Coca-Cola. Stir frequently and bring to a boil.

4. Pour over dry ingredients (sugar, flour, marshmallows), blending well.

5. In a separate bowl, combine: baking soda and buttermilk, then eggs and vanilla. Whisk briefly, then fold in to batter, mixing well.

6. Pour in to a greased 13'x9' pan (I use aluminum) and bake for 35-45 minutes, I typically set the timer for 40 min's.

7. While cake is baking, begin making icing (recipe below). Once cake is ready, remove from oven. Delicately prick holes in to cake (using a toothpick), then ice immediately. This will allow the icing to seep in to the cake's crevices.

Icing

1. In a saucepan, combine: butter, cocoa and Coca-Cola. Stir frequently and bring to a boil.

2. In a separate bowl, add confectioner's sugar. Pour boiled ingredients over confectioner's sugar and blend well.

3. Add vanilla extract and continue to mix until icing is smooth and free of clumps. Evenly spread over hot cake.

4. *When cake has cooled, cut in to squares and serve.
    Cake can be stored in or out of fridge, covered

20. Celeriac Soup with Crispy Shiitakes

Prep time: 15 minutes

Cook time: 40 minutes

Total Time: 55 minutes

Makes about: 6 servings

Ingredient:

- 3 tablespoons extra-virgin olive oil
- 1 large leek, white part only, rinsed and diced
- 2 celery stalks, diced
- Sea salt
- 2 cloves garlic, minced
- 2 pounds celery root (celeriac), peeled and diced
- 1 fennel bulb, diced
- 6 cups Magic Mineral Broth
- 1 tablespoon freshly squeezed lemon juice
- ¼ teaspoon Grade B maple syrup
- 1 cup Crispy Shiitakes, for garnish

Directions:

1. Heat the olive oil in a soup pot over medium heat, then add the leek, celery, and ¼ teaspoon salt. Sauté

until the vegetables begin to get tender, about 6 minutes. Add the garlic and cook for another 30 seconds, then stir in the celery root, fennel, and another ¼ teaspoon salt. Sauté about 5 minutes more, stirring often. Pour in ½ cup of the broth to deglaze the pot, stirring to loosen any bits stuck to the bottom, and cook until the liquid is reduced by half.

2. Add the remaining 5½ cups of broth and another ¼ teaspoon salt. Bring the soup to a boil, then reduce the heat to medium, cover, and simmer until the vegetables are tender, about 20 to 25 minutes.

3. In a blender, puree the soup in batches until very smooth, each time adding the cooking liquid first and then the celery root mixture, and adding additional liquid, as needed. Pour the soup back into the pot, heat gently, and stir in the lemon juice. Taste; you may want to add a pinch more salt. Serve garnished with the mushrooms or store in an airtight container in the refrigerator for up to 5 days or in the freezer for up to 3 months.

DINNER

21. Orange Pistachio Quinoa

Prep Time: 15 Minutes

 Cook Time: 15 Minutes

Total Time: 30 Minutes

 Makes 6 Servings

Ingredient:

- 1/2 cup raw pistachios
- 1 1/2 cups quinoa
- 2 1/2 cups Magic Mineral Broth or water
- 1 teaspoon sea salt
- 1 teaspoon cumin
- 1/2 teaspoon coriander
- 1/8 teaspoon freshly ground pepper
- 1/2 cup chopped fresh mint
- 2 scallions, both green and white parts, finely chopped
- 1/8 cup freshly squeezed orange juice
- Zest of 1 orange
- 1 1/2 tablespoons olive oil
- 1 1/2 tablespoons freshly squeezed lemon juice

- 1/2 cup raisins

Directions:

1. Spread the pistachios in an even layer on a sheet pan and bake for 7 to 10 minutes, until aromatic and slightly browned. Let cool.

2. Place the quinoa in a fine-mesh strainer and rinse well under cold running water to remove all the resin.

3. In a pot, bring the broth and 1 teaspoon salt to a boil. Add the quinoa and cover. Decrease the heat and simmer for 15 minutes. Transfer from the heat and fluff with a fork. Spread mixture out on a sheet pan and "rake" with a fork occasionally until cooled.

4. Transfer the quinoa from the sheet pan to a large bowl. Stir in the cumin, coriander, salt, and pepper. Add the mint, scallions, orange juice, orange zest, olive oil, lemon juice, toasted pistachios, and raisins. Mix well and taste; you may need a pinch of salt, a squeeze of lemon, or a dash of olive oil.

22. Mediterranean Lentil Salad

Prep Time: 10 Minutes

 Cook Time: 25 Minutes

Total Time: 35 minutes

Makes 6 Servings

Ingredient:

- 1 cup dried lentils, French Le Puy
- 2 bay leaves
- 1 clove garlic, peeled and bruised
- 1/4 teaspoon dried oregano
- 1 cinnamon stick
- 1/4 teaspoon sea salt (used during the cooking of the lentils)
- 1/4 cup extra virgin olive oil
- 3 tablespoons lemon juice
- 1 teaspoon lemon zest
- 1/2teaspoon ground cumin
- 1/2teaspoon sea salt
- 1 medium red bell pepper, seeded and finely diced
- 1 small cucumber, seeded and diced small
- 1/4 cup Kalamata olives, rinsed and sliced

- 3 tablespoons chopped mint
- 3 tablespoons chopped parsley
- 2 ounces feta cheese, (optional)

Directions:

1. Rinse the lentils well and place in a saucepan with bay leaves, 1 bruised garlic clove, oregano and cinnamon stick. Cover with water or broth by 2 inches and a generous pinch of sea salt. Bring to a boil, reduce the heat to low, add the sea salt and simmer until the lentils are tender, 20-25 minutes. Drain. In a small bowl whisk together the olive oil, lemon juice, zest,cumin and salt in a small bowl. Toss the vinaigrette with the lentils, red bell pepper, cucumbers, olives, feta cheese if using, mint and parsley in a mixing bowl. Transfer to a large serving bowl or individual plates and serve at room temperature.

23. Poached Eggs with Basil Lemon Drizzle

Prep Time 2 Minutes

 Cook Time 5 Minutes

Total Time: 7 minutes

Make about: Serves 4

Ingerdient:

- 1 tablespoon vinegar
- 4 organic eggs
- Sea salt

Directions:

1. Pour 6 inches of water into a large saucepan and place over medium-high heat. When it's almost boiling, add the vinegar, then crack each egg open in a small dish and gently slide the egg in the water. Maintain the water temperature at just below a simmer, turning the heat down to low if necessary. Cook until the egg whites are set and the centers are still soft, about 3 minutes. Remove with a slotted spoon and place on a paper towel to drain off excess water.

2. Serve immediately, sprinkling each egg with a pinch of sea salt and topping with 2 teaspoons of Basil Lemon Drizzle.

24. Simple Scrambled Eggs with kale

Prep Time 10 Minutes

Cook Time 5 Minutes

Total Time: 15 minutes

Makes about 2 Servings

Ingredient:

- 4 organic eggs
- 1/4 teaspoon sea salt
- 1 teaspoon turmeric (optional)
- 1/4 teaspoon freshly ground pepper
- 1 tablespoon water
- 2 teaspoons olive oil
- 1 cup kale, stemmed and chopped into bite-sized pieces

Directions:

1. In a medium bowl, crack the eggs, then add the salt, turmeric, pepper, and water and beat well with a whisk or fork until the egg mixture becomes foamy.

2. Heat a 10-inch skillet over medium heat, then add the olive oil. When the olive oil begins to shimmer, add

the egg mixture and turn down the heat to medium-low. Add the eggs to the pan and cook, stirring frequently with a wooden spoon. After a minute or two, the eggs will begin to form curds. Add the greens and keep stirring continuously until the eggs are soft and shiny. Remove the mixture from the heat and serve immediately.

25. Curried Deviled Eggs

Prep Time 15 Minutes

 Cook Time 20 Minutes

Total Time: 35 miuntes

Makes about: 4 Servings

Ingredient:

- 4 organic eggs
- 2 tablespoons organic plain yogurt
- 1 tablespoon chopped fresh cilantro
- 2 teaspoons chopped fresh mint
- 1/2 teaspoon curry powder
- 1/4 teaspoon turmeric
- 1/4 teaspoon freshly ground black pepper
- 1/4 teaspoon sea salt

Directions:

1. Put the eggs in saucepan and add enough cold water to cover them by about 1 inch. Bring to a boil over medium-high heat, then cover and immediately remove

2. from the heat. Let sit for 15 to 18 minutes, until the water is tepid.

3. Transfer the eggs to a bowl of cool water. When they're cool enough to handle, peel them under cold running water. Cut the eggs in half lengthwise. Scoop

4. out the yolks and put them in a small bowl. Add the yogurt, cilantro, 1 teaspoon of the mint, curry powder, turmeric, pepper, and salt and stir with a fork until

5. smooth. Spoon the mixture into the egg whites and sprinkle with the remaining mint.

Prep Time: 25 Minutes

Cook Time: 45 Minutes

Total Time: 1hour 10 minutes

Makes about 4 Servings

Ingredients:

Squash:

- 4 acorn squash
- 2 tablespoons extra-virgin olive oil
- ¼ teaspoon sea salt
- ¼ teaspoon ground allspice
- ¼ teaspoon ground ginger
- ¼ teaspoon ground cinnamon
- Pinch of red pepper flakes

Filling

- 1 cup quinoa
- 1 tablespoon plus 2 teaspoons extra-virgin olive oil
- 1 tablespoon finely diced shallot
- 3 tablespoons finely diced fennel

- ¼ teaspoon ground cumin

- ¼ teaspoon ground coriander

- 2 cups Magic Mineral Broth or water

- ½ teaspoon sea salt

- 2 cloves garlic, minced

- Pinch of red pepper flakes

- ½ cup dried cranberries or raisins

- 6 cups stemmed and chopped Swiss chard or kale, in bite-size pieces

- Fresh squeezed lemon juice

Directions:

1. Preheat the oven to 350°F and line a sheet pan with parchment paper.

2. To make the squash, cut the tops off the squash and scoop out the strings and seeds. Also cut the pointy ends off the bottoms of the squash so they'll stand up once they're stuffed.

3. Stir the olive oil, salt, allspice, ginger, cinnamon, and red pepper flakes together in a bowl. Use a brush to spread the spice mixture over the inside of the squash. Place the squash, top side down, on the prepared pan and roast for 20 to 25 minutes, until tender. Check

after 20 minutes by touching the top of a squash with your finger. If it's soft, transfer the squash from the oven and cover with foil until you're ready to fill them.

4. Meanwhile, make the filling. Put the quinoa in a fine-mesh sieve and rinse well under running cold water.

5. Heat the 2 teaspoons of olive oil in a saucepan over medium heat. Add the shallot and fennel and sauté until soft, about 3 minutes. Stir in the cumin and coriander, then stir in the quinoa. Stir in the broth and 1/4 teaspoon of the salt, cover, and bring to a boil, then lower the heat and simmer for 15 to 20 minutes, until the quinoa has absorbed all of the liquid. Remove from the heat, and fluff with a fork.

6. While the quinoa is cooking, heat the 1 tablespoon of olive oil in a large sauté pan over medium heat, then add the garlic, red pepper flakes, and cranberries. Stir for 10 seconds, then add the kale and the remaining 1/4 teaspoon salt. Sauté until the greens are tender, about 5 minutes for kale, or 3 minutes for chard.

Remove from the heat and stir in a squeeze of the lemon juice.

7. To assemble the dish, spoon the quinoa mixture into the squash, then top each squash with a scoop of the greens.

27. High-Flying Turkey Black Bean Chili

Prep Time: 20 Minutes

Cook Time: 35 MinutesTotal

Time: 55 minutes

Makes about 6 Servings

Ingredient:

- 3 tablespoons extra-virgin olive oil
- 1 large yellow onion, chopped
- 1 large clove garlic, minced
- 1 jalapeño, deribbed, seeded, and minced
- 2 teaspoons chili powder
- 1 teaspoon ancho chile powder
- 1 teaspoon smoked paprika
- 1 heaping teaspoon ground cumin
- 1 teaspoon dried oregano, gently crushed in your hand
- 1/2 heaping teaspoon ground cinnamon
- 1 pound ground white or dark turkey meat, or a combination
- 1 (28-ounce) can crushed tomatoes
- 2 red bell peppers, chopped into bite-size pieces

- 4 cups cooked black beans or 2 (15-ounce) cans, rinsed
- 1 tablespoon Grade B maple syrup
- Freshly squeezed lime juice

Cilantro Avocado Cream (Optional)

- 1 avocado, halved and flesh scooped out
- 2 tablespoons water
- 3/4 teaspoon freshly squeezed lime juice
- 2 teaspoons coarsely chopped fresh cilantro
- 1/4 teaspoon sea salt

Directions:

1. In a bowl, combine the drained, rinsed beans with a spritz of lime juice and a pinch of salt; set aside. In a 6-quart pot, heat the olive oil over medium heat. Add the onions and a pinch of salt and sauté for 3 minutes, until the onions are translucent. Add the garlic, jalapeño, chili powder, ancho chile powder, paprika, cumin, oregano, and cinnamon and sauté for another minute. Add the turkey and 1/4 teaspoon of salt, breaking up the meat with a wooden spoon, and brown for about 3 minutes. If the pan is dry or the spices stick, pour in a little juice from the tomatoes to

deglaze the pan, stirring with the wooden spoon to loosen any bits stuck to the pan. Add the tomatoes and another pinch of salt, then the peppers and beans and another pinch of salt. Stir to combine. Bring it to a simmer over medium low heat, then cover and simmer for 20 minutes, stirring occasionally.

2. Remove the cover and simmer for 10 minutes more, stirring occasionally. Stir in the maple syrup. Taste, and add lime juice and salt as needed.

3. To make the cilantro avocado cream (which is an optional garnish), put the avocado, water, lime juice, cilantro, and salt in a blender and process until very smooth, about 1 minute. Transfer to a small bowl.

28. Silk Road Pumpkin Soup

Prep time: 15 minutes

 Cook time: 45 minutes

Total Time:1 hour

Makes about 6 servings

Ingredient:

- ¼ teaspoon ground allspice
- ½ teaspoon ground cinnamon
- ½ teaspoon ground cardamom
- 2½ pounds kabocha squash, quartered and seeded
- 1 yellow onion, diced
- 2 parsnips, diced small
- 2 cloves garlic, minced
- 1 tablespoon minced fresh ginger
- 6 cups Magic Mineral Broth, plus more if needed

Directions:

1. Preheat the oven to 400°F. Line a baking sheet with parchment paper.

2. In a small bowl combine 2 tablespoons of the olive oil, ¼ teaspoon salt, the allspice, ¼ teaspoon of the cinnamon, and ¼ teaspoon of the cardamom. Rub the spice mixture into the cut sides of the squash using your hands or a pastry brush. Place the seasoned squash on the prepared baking sheet and roast for 30 minutes, or until tender when pierced with a knife.

3. While the squash is roasting, heat the remaining 2 tablespoons of olive oil in a soup pot over medium-high heat, then add the onion, parsnips, and ¼ teaspoon salt and sauté until golden and translucent, about 6 minutes. Add the remaining ¼ teaspoon of cinnamon, the remaining ¼ teaspoon of cardamom, and the garlic and ginger and sauté until fragrant, about 30 seconds more. Pour in 1 cup of the broth to deglaze the pot, stirring to loosen any bits stuck to the bottom. Remove from the heat and set aside. When the squash has cooled to the touch, scoop

4. the flesh into the pot with the vegetable mixture.

29. Pastured Beef Bone Broth

Prep Time: 25 Minutes

 Cook Time: 8 To 24 Hours

makes about 6 serving

Ingerdients:

- 3 pounds marrow bones from grass-fed organic beef
- 6 unpeeled carrots, cut into thirds
- 2 unpeeled yellow onions, quartered
- 1 leek, white and green parts, cut into thirds
- 1 bunch celery, including the heart, cut into thirds
- 5 unpeeled cloves garlic, halved
- ½ bunch fresh flat-leaf parsley
- 4 unpeeled red potatoes, quartered
- 2 unpeeled Japanese or regular sweet potatoes, quartered
- 1 unpeeled garnet yam (sweet potato), quartered
- 1 (8-inch) strip of kombu
- 2 bay leaves
- 12 black peppercorns
- 4 whole allspice or juniper berries
- 1 tablespoon apple cider vinegar
- 8 quarts cold, filtered water, plus more if needed

- 1 teaspoon sea salt

Directions:

1. Rinse all of the vegetables well, including the kombu. In a 12-quart or larger stockpot, combine the bones, carrots, onions, leek, celery, garlic, parsley, red potatoes, sweet potatoes, yam, kombu, bay leaves, peppercorns, allspice berries, and vinegar. Pour in the water, cover, and bring to a boil over high heat. Remove the lid, decrease the heat to low, and skim off the scum that has risen to the top. Simmer gently, partially covered, for 8 to 24 hours. As the broth simmers, some of the water will evaporate; add more if the vegetables begin to peek out.

2. Remove and discard the bones, then strain the broth through a large, coarse-mesh sieve. Stir in the salt. Let cool to room temperature, and then refrigerate overnight in an airtight container.

3. Skim off as much fat as you can from the top of the broth, then portion into airtight containers.

4. Store in the refrigerator for up to 5 days or in the freezer for up to 6 months.

30. Wendy's Wunderbar

Prep Time: 25 minutes

Cook Time: 1 hour for chilling

Total Time: 1 hour 25 minutes

Makes about 16 servings

Ingredients:

- 2 oz. dark chocolate (60 to 72% cacao content), finely chopped
- 1 oz. unsweetened baking chocolate, finely chopped
- ⅓ c. shelled pistachios
- ⅓ c. almonds, toasted
- 8 oz. Medjool dates, halved and pitted
- ½ tsp. vanilla extract
- ⅛ tsp. sea salt
- ⅓ c. dried cherries

Directions:

1. Line an 8-inch square pan with two pieces of waxed paper long enough to overlap on all four sides. Lightly oil the waxed paper, then line the bottom with another piece. Put the chocolate in a heatproof bowl and set over a saucepan of simmering water. Heat, stirring

often, just until the chocolate is melted and smooth.
Remove from the heat.

2. Put the pistachios and almonds in food processor and
    pulse three or four times to coarsely chop. Add the
    dates, melted chocolate, vanilla, and salt. Pulse until
    the ingredients begin to hold together, almost like
    dough. Add the cherries and pulse a few more times,
    until the cherries are coarsely chopped and evenly
    distributed. Transfer to the prepared pan and press in
    an even layer using your hands. Smooth the top with a
    spatula. Cover with a piece of parchment or waxed
    paper and chill until firm, about 1 hour.

3. Remove from the pan by lifting the edges of the waxed
    paper, and place on a cutting board, still atop the
    waxed paper. Using an oiled knife to prevent sticking,
    cut into 16 squares. Put the bars in a container, with
    waxed paper between the layers if stacked, or wrap
    the bars individually in foil. Store in the refrigerator
    or freezer. Warm to room temperature before eating.

www.ingramcontent.com/pod-product-compliance
Lightning Source LLC
Chambersburg PA
CBHW061333120726

48001CB00002B/837